C000051056

Your Plant-Based Lunch Cookbook

Amazing Plant-Based Recipes to Boost Your Lunch and Manage Your Weight

Dave Ingram

© Copyright 2020 - All rights reserved.

The content contained within this book may not be reproduced, duplicated or transmitted without direct written permission from the author or the publisher.

Under no circumstances will any blame or legal responsibility be held against the publisher, or author, for any damages, reparation, or monetary loss due to the information contained within this book. Either directly or indirectly.

Legal Notice:

This book is copyright protected. This book is only for personal use. You cannot amend, distribute, sell, use, quote or paraphrase any part, or the content within this book, without the consent of the author or publisher.

Disclaimer Notice:

Please note the information contained within this document is for educational and entertainment purposes only. All effort has been executed to present accurate, up to date, and reliable, complete information. No warranties of any kind are declared or implied. Readers acknowledge that the author is not engaging in the rendering of legal, financial, medical or professional advice. The content within this book has been derived from various sources. Please consult a licensed professional before attempting any techniques outlined in this book.

By reading this document, the reader agrees that under no circumstances is the author responsible for any losses, direct or indirect, which are incurred as a result of the use of information contained within this document, including, but not limited to, — errors, omissions, or inaccuracies.

Table of contents

Cashew-Ginger Soba Noodle Bowl

Total time: 25 minutes

Ingredients

For the Bowls

7 ounces noodles

1 carrot, julienned

1 bell pepper,

1 cup peas, trimmed and sliced

2 tbsp scallions

1   cup kale or lettuce

1 avocado,

2   tablespoons cashews, chopped

For the Dressing

1   tablespoon grated fresh ginger

2   tablespoons cashew butter, or almond or sunflower seed butter 2 tablespoons rice vinegar

2 tbsp tamari or soy sauce

1 teaspoon toasted sesame oil

2 to 3 tablespoons water (optional)

Directions

1.	Add water to the noodles. Add cool water if necessary. The soba will take 6 to 7 minutes to cook, and you can occasionally stir. Rinse with hot or cold water, depending on whether you want a hot or cold bowl.

2.	You can have the vegetables raw. If you'd like to cook them, sauté the carrot withwater, broth, olive oil. Add the bell pepper, the peas and scallions to warm for a minute before turning off the heat.

3.	Whisk together all the ingredients, or puréeing in a small blender, adding 2 to 3 tbsp of water to make a creamy consistency. Set aside.

4.	Arrange your bowl, starting with a layer of chopped kale or spinach

5.	Top with the dressing, sliced avocado, and a sprinkle of chopped cashews.

Mediterranean Hummus Pizza

Total time: 40 minutes

Ingredients

½ zucchini, thinly sliced

½ red onion, thinly sliced

1   cup cherry tomatoes, halved

2   to 4 tablespoons pitted and chopped black olives
Pinch sea salt

Drizzle olive oil (optional) 2 prebaked pizza crusts

½ cup Classic Hummus, or Roasted Red Pepper
Hummus 2 to 4 tablespoons Cheesy Sprinkle

Directions

1.   Preheat the oven to 400°F.

2.   Place the zucchini, onion, cherry tomatoes, and
olives in a large bowl, sprinkle them with the sea salt

and toss them a bit. Drizzle with oil (if using) to seal in the flavor and keep them from drying out in the oven.

3.   Lay the two crusts out on a large baking sheet. Spread half the hummus on each crust, and top with the veggie mixture and some Cheesy Sprinkle.

4.   Pop the pizzas in the oven for 20 to 30 minutes or until the veggies are soft.

5.   Make Ahead: For a shortcut, lightly sauté the veggies before putting them on the pizza, so you only have to bake it for a few minutes until warmed through. You could even use some leftover sautéed vegetables.

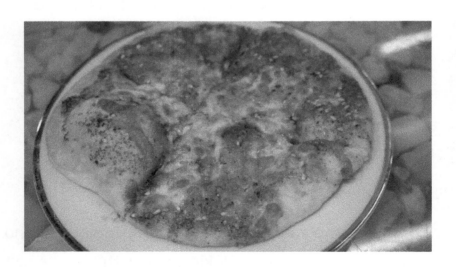

Maple Dijon Burgers

Total time: 50 minutes

Ingredients

1 red bell pepper

1   (19-ounce) can chickpeas, rinsed and drained, or 2 cups cooked 1 cup ground almonds

2   teaspoons Dijon mustard 2 teaspoons maple syrup

1 garlic clove, pressed Juice of ½ lemon

1 teaspoon dried oregano

½ teaspoon dried sage 1 cup spinach

1 to 1½ cups rolled oats

Directions

1.   Preheat the oven to 350°F. Cover baking sheet with parchment paper.

2.	Cut the red pepper in half, remove the stem and seeds, and put on the baking sheet cut side up in the oven. Roast in the oven.

3.	Put the chickpeas in the food processor, along with the almonds, mustard, maple syrup, garlic, lemon juice, oregano, sage, and spinach. Pulse until things are thoroughly combined but not puréed. When the red pepper is softened a bit, about 10 minutes, add it to the processor along with the oats and pulse until they are chopped just enough to form patties.

4.	If you don't have a food processor, mash the chickpeas with a potato masher or fork, and make sure everything else is chopped up as finely as possible, then stir together.

5.	Scoop up ¼-cup portions and form into 12 patties, and lay them out on the baking sheet.

6.	Put the burgers in the oven and bake until the outside is lightly browned for about 30 minutes.

Cajun Burgers

Total time: 55 minutes

Ingredients

For the Dressing

1 tablespoon tahini

1 tablespoon apple cider vinegar 2 teaspoons Dijon mustard

1 to 2 tablespoons water

1 to 2 garlic cloves, pressed 1 teaspoon dried basil

1   teaspoon dried thyme

½ teaspoon dried oregano

½ teaspoon dried sage

½ teaspoon smoked paprika

¼ teaspoon cayenne pepper

¼ teaspoon sea salt

Pinch freshly ground black pepper

For the Burgers

2   cups water

1   cup kasha (toasted buckwheat) Pinch sea salt

2   carrots, grated

Handful fresh parsley, chopped 1 teaspoon olive oil (optional)

Directions

For the Dressing

1.   In a medium bowl, whisk together the tahini, vinegar, and mustard until the mixture is very thick. Add 1 and half tbsp water to thin it out, and whisk again until smooth.

2.   Stir in the rest of the ingredients. Set aside for the flavors to blend.

For the Burgers

1.   Put the water, buckwheat, and sea salt in a medium pot. Let boil for 2 and half minutes, then turn down to low, cover, and simmer for 15 minutes. Buckwheat is fully cooked when it is soft, and no liquid

is left at the bottom of the pot. Do not stir the buckwheat while it is cooking.

2.   Once the buckwheat is cooked, transfer it to a large bowl. Stir the grated carrot, fresh parsley, and all the dressing into the buckwheat. Scoop up ¼-cup portions and form into patties.

3.   You can either panfry or bake the burgers. To panfry, heat a large skillet to medium, add 1 teaspoon olive oil, and cook the burgers for about 5 minutes on the first side. Flip, and cook for another 5 minutes. Bake at 330°F for 30 minutes.

Grilled Seitan in Barbeque Sauce

Total time: 10 minutes

Ingredients

8 oz of seitan (thinly sliced or chopped in 1" chunks)

½ cup of barbecue sauce

Cubed vegetable of your choice (blanch)

Directions

1.   To start, make sure to soak the skewers in the water to prevent burning.

2.   Put seitan in a plastic bag or cover well with barbecue sauce in a

3.   deep pan. Mix and allow marinating for at least an hour; much better if longer.

4.   Heat a grill to medium-high temperature.

5.   Meanwhile, thread the seitan and vegetables on the skewers alternately. Grill the skewers until the

seitan is cooked and golden brown on both sides while brushing with barbecue sauce.

6.   Dish with the food and service.

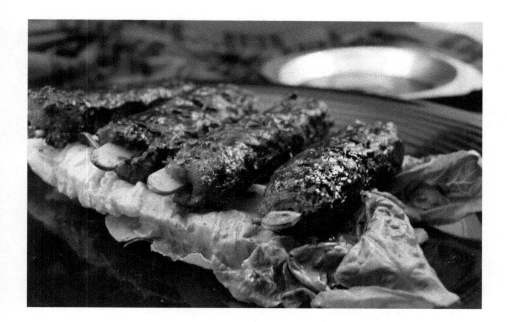

Tofu Wraps Curried

Total time: 25 minutes

Ingredients

½ cup garden greens of your choice (shredded) 3 tbsp of mint sauce

4 tbsp of yogurt (non-dairy, heaped) 3 pcs of 200g of tofu (cut in 15 cubes) 2 tbsp of tandoori curry paste

2 tbsp of oil

2 large cloves of garlic (sliced) 2 small size of onions (sliced) 8 chapatis (whole-wheat)

2 pcs of limes (cut into quarters)

Directions

1.   In a medium bowl, combine the garden greens, mint sauce, yogurt, and set aside.

2.   In a medium bowl, mix the tofu, tandoori paste, and oil.

3. Heat a skillet over medium temperature and cook the tofu until cooked within. Stir in the garlic, onions, and cook for 3 more minutes. Turn the heat off.

4. Toast the chapatis in a preheated grill pan until golden brown and lay on a flat surface.

5. Spoon in the garden green mixture, top with the tofu mix, wrap, and serve warm.

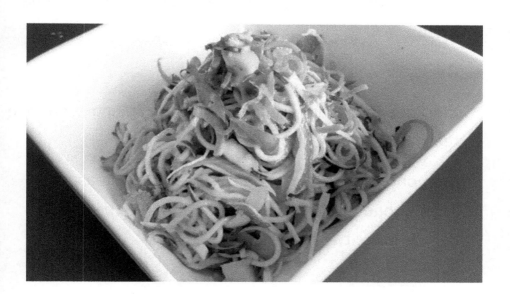

Green Pea Fritter

Preparation Time: 10 minutes

Cooking Time: 20 minutes

Servings: 10

Ingredients:

Frozen peas, two cups

Olive oil, one tablespoon + one tablespoon Onion, one diced

Garlic, three tablespoons

Chickpea four, one- and one-half cups Baking soda, one teaspoon

Salt, one quarter teaspoon Rosemary, one teaspoon Thyme, one half teaspoon Marjoram, one teaspoon Lemon juice, two tablespoons

Directions:

1.	Heat the oven to 350. Use spray oil to spray a baking sheet. Boil the peas for five minutes.

2.	Pour one tablespoon of olive oil in a skillet and fry the garlic and onion for five minutes.

3.	Pour the garlic and onion with the olive oil in a bowl and add the cooked peas, mashing them until they make a thick paste. Blend in the marjoram, thyme, rosemary, salt, baking soda, and chickpea flour.

4.	Dampen your hands and form the mash into ten equal-sized patties. Brush the patties with the other tablespoon of olive oil.

5.	Bake them for eighteen minutes in the oven, turning them over after nine minutes.

Nutrition: calories 224 fat 3 carbs 14 protein 6

Roasted Mushrooms and Shallots

Preparation Time: 10 minutes

Cooking Time: 20 minutes

Servings: 4

Ingredients:

Mushrooms, fresh, one-pound cut into bite-size pieces Shallots, two cups sliced thick

Olive oil, two tablespoons Thyme, dried, one teaspoon salt, one quarter teaspoon

Black pepper, one-quarter teaspoon Red wine vinegar, one third cup

Directions:

Place the shallots and mushrooms in a large bowl and add salt, pepper, thyme, and olive oil and toss the ingredients together to coat the shallots and mushrooms thoroughly.

Roast the veggies on a baking sheet for fifteen minutes. Pour the red wine vinegar over the veggies and bake for five more minutes.

Nutrition: calories 178 fat 7 carbs 23 protein 5

Garlic Chili Roasted Kohlrabi

Preparation Time: 5 minutes

Cooking Time: 12 minutes

Servings: 1

Ingredients:

Olive oil, two tablespoons Garlic, minced, one tablespoon Chili pepper, one teaspoon salt, one quarter teaspoon

Kohlrabi, one and one-half pounds, peel and cut into one half inch wedges

Cilantro, fresh, chopped, two tablespoons

Directions:

1.   Heat your oven to 450. Put in the kohlrabi and toss well to coat the kohlrabi.

2.   Bake the coated kohlrabi for twenty minutes, stirring it around when you are about halfway done with cooking. Sprinkle on the cilantro and serve.

Vegetarian Nachos

Preparation Time: 15 minutes

Cooking Time: 0 minutes

Servings: 6

Ingredients:

Pita chips, whole wheat, three cups Nutritional yeast, one half cup Oregano, dried, one tablespoon minced Romaine lettuce, one cup chopped

Grape tomatoes, one-half cup cut in quarters Olive oil, two tablespoons

Lemon juice, one tablespoon Hummus, one-third cup prepared Black pepper, one half teaspoon Red onion, two tablespoons minced

Tofu, one-half cup cut into small crumbles Black olives, two tablespoons chopped

Directions:

1.   Mix the hummus, pepper, olive oil, and lemon juice in a mixing bowl. Spread a layer of the pita chips on a serving platter.

2.   Drizzle three-fourths of the hummus mix over the pita chips. Use lettuce, red onion, tomatoes, and olives to garnish the hummus.

3.   Make a small mound of the leftover hummus in the middle of the chips, then garnish it all with the oregano and the nutritional yeast.

Nutrition: calories 159 fat 10 carbs 13 protein 4

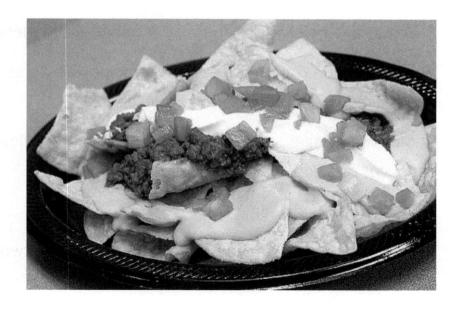

Vegan Macaroni and Cheese

Preparation Time: 15 minutes

Cooking Time: 20 minutes

Servings: 4

Ingredients:

Elbow macaroni, whole grain, eight ounces, cooked
Nutritional yeast, one quarter cup

Garlic, minced, two tablespoons Apple cider vinegar,
two teaspoons

Broccoli, one head with florets cut into bite-sized pieces

Water, one cup (more if needed), Garlic powder, one
half teaspoon Avocado oil, two tablespoons

Red pepper, flakes, one eighth teaspoon Onion, yellow,
chopped, one cup

Salt, one half teaspoon

Russet potato, peeled and grated, one cup (about two
small potatoes)

Dry mustard powder, one half teaspoon Onion powder, one half teaspoon

Directions:

1. Cook the broccoli for five minutes in boiling water. Add the cooked broccoli to the cooked pasta in a large mixing bowl.

2. Cook the onion in the avocado oil for five minutes, then stir in the red pepper flakes, garlic, salt, mustard powder, garlic powder, grated potato, and onion powder. Cook this for three minutes and then pour in the water and mix well. Cook this for eight to ten minutes or until the potatoes are soft.

3. Pour all of this mixture carefully into a blender and add in the nutritional yeast and the vinegar and then blend. When this is creamy and smooth, pour it into the mixing bowl and mix well with the broccoli and pasta.

Nutrition: calories 506 fat 22 carbs 67 protein 18

Cilantro Lime Coleslaw

Preparation Time: 5 minutes

Cooking Time: 0 minutes

Servings: 5

Ingredients:

Avocados, two

Garlic, minced, one tablespoon

Coleslaw, ready-made in a bag, fourteen ounces
Cilantro, fresh leaves, one-quarter cup minced

Salt, one half teaspoon Lime juice, two tablespoons
Water, one quarter cup

Directions:

1.   Except for the slaw mix, but all of the ingredients are listed in a blender. Blend these ingredients well until they are creamy and smooth.

2.   Mix the coleslaw mix in with this dressing, and then toss it gently to mix it well.

3.   Keep the mixed coleslaw in the refrigerator until you are ready to serve.

Nutrition: calories 119 fat 3 carbs 3 protein 3

Black-Eyed Peas and Corn Salad

Preparation Time: 30 minutes

Cooking Time: 50 minutes

Servings: 4

Ingredients:

2½ cups cooked black-eyed peas 3 ears corn, kernels removed

1 medium ripe tomato, diced

½ medium red onion, peeled and diced small

½ pepper, deseeded

1 jalapeño pepper, deseeded and minced

½ cup finely chopped cilantro

¼ cup plus 2 tablespoons balsamic vinegar 3 cloves garlic, peeled and minced

1 teaspoon toasted and ground cumin seeds

Directions:

1.   Stir together all the ingredients in a large bowl and refrigerate for about 1 hour, or until well chilled.

2.   Serve chilled.

Nutrition:

Calories: 247 Fat: 1.8g Carbs: 47.6g Protein: 12.9g Fiber: 11.7g

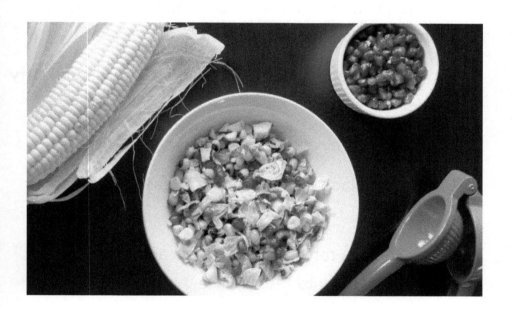

Indian Tomato and Garbanzo Stew

Preparation Time: 15 minutes

Cooking Time: 50 minutes

Servings: 4 to 6

Ingredients:

1   large onion, quartered and thinly sliced 1-inch fresh ginger, peeled and minced

2   cloves garlic, peeled and minced 1 teaspoon curry powder

1 teaspoon cumin seeds

1 teaspoon black mustard seeds 1 teaspoon coriander seeds,

1½ lb. (680 g) tomatoes, deseeded and puréed 1 red bell pepper, cut into ½-inch dice

1 green bell pepper, cut into ½-inch dice 3 cups cooked garbanzo beans

1 tablespoon garam masala 1/3 cup water

Directions:

1.   Heat the water in a medium saucepan over medium-low heat. Add the onion, ginger, garlic, curry powder, and seeds to the pan. Sauté for about 10 minutes, or until the onion is tender, stirring frequently.

2.   Add the tomatoes and simmer for 9 minutes. Add the peppers and garbanzo beans. Reduce heat. Cover and for 32 minutes, stirring occasionally. Stir in the garam masala and serve.

Nutrition:

Calories: 100 Fat: 1.2g Carbs: 20.9g Protein: 5.1g Fiber: 7.0g

Simple Baked Navy Beans

Preparation Time: 10 minutes

Cooking Time: 2½ to 3 hours

Servings: 8

Ingredients:

1½ cups navy beans 8 cups water

1 bay leaf

½ cup finely chopped green bell pepper

½ cup onion

1 tsp minced garlic

½ cup unsweetened tomato purée 3 tablespoons molasses

1 tablespoon fresh lemon juice

Directions:

1.   Put oven to 320ºF (150ºC).

2.   Place beans and water in a pot, along with the bay leaf, green pepper, onion, and garlic. Cover and cook for 1½ to 2 hours, or until the beans are softened. Remove from the heat and drain, reserving the cooking liquid. Discard the bay leaf.

3.   Transfer the mixture to a casserole dish with a cover. Stir in the remaining ingredients and 1 cup of the reserved cooking liquid. Bake in the oven for 1 hour, covered. Stir occasionally during baking and add a little more cooking liquid if needed to keep the beans moist.

4.   Serve warm.

Nutrition:

Calories: 162 Fat: 0.6g Carbs: 31.3g Protein: 9.1g Fiber: 6.4g

Vinegary Black Beans

Preparation Time: 10 minutes

Cooking Time: 2 hours

Servings: 8

Ingredients:

1 pound (454 g) black beans, soaked overnight and drained 10½ cups water, divided

1 green pepper, cut in half

1 onion, finely chopped

1 green bell pepper, finely chopped

4 cloves garlic, pressed

1 tablespoon maple syrup (optional) 1 tablespoon Mrs. Dash seasoning 1 bay leaf

¼ teaspoon dried oregano 2 tablespoons cider vinegar

Directions:

1.	Place the beans, 10 cups of water, and green bell pepper in a large pot. Cook over medium heat for about 45 minutes or until the green pepper is tendered. Remove the green pepper and discard.

2.	Meanwhile, in a different pot, combine the onion, chopped green pepper, garlic, and the remaining ½ cup of the water. Sauté for 13 minutes, or until soft.

3.	Add 1 and half cup of the cooked beans to the pot with vegetables. Mash the beans and vegetables with a potato masher. Add to the pot with the beans, maple syrup (if desired), Mrs. Dash, bay leaf, and oregano. Cover and cook over low heat for 1 hour.

4.	Drizzle in the vinegar and continue to cook for another hour.

5.	Serve warm.

Nutrition:

Calories: 226 Fat: 0.9g Carbs: 42.7g Protein: 12.9g Fiber: 9.9g

Spiced Lentil Burgers

Preparation Time: 10 minutes

Cooking Time: 43 minutes

Servings: 4

Ingredients:

¼ cup minced onion 1 clove garlic, minced 2 tablespoons water

1   cup chopped boiled potatoes 1 cup cooked lentils

2   tablespoons minced fresh parsley 1 teaspoon onion powder

1 teaspoon minced fresh basil 1 teaspoon dried dill

1 teaspoon paprika

Directions:

1.   Preheat the oven to 350ºF.

2.   In a pot, sauté the onion and garlic in the water for about 3 minutes, or until soft.

3.   Combine the lentils and potatoes in a large bowl and mash together well. Add the cooked onion and garlic and the remaining ingredients to the lentil-potato mixture and stir until well combined.

4.   Form the mixture into four patties and place it on a nonstick baking sheet. Bake in the oven for 20 minutes. Turnover and bake for an additional 20 minutes.

5.   Serve hot.

Nutrition:

Calories: 101 Fat: 0.4g Carbs: 19.9g Protein: 5.5g Fiber: 5.3g

Pecan-Maple Granola

Preparation Time: 5 minutes

Cooking Time: 50 minutes

Servings: 4

Ingredients:

1½ cups rolled oats

¼ cup maple syrup (optional)

¼ cup pecan pieces

1 teaspoon vanilla extract

½ teaspoon ground cinnamon

Directions:

1.   Preheat the oven to 300ºF. Line a baking sheet with parchment paper.

2.   Stir all the ingredients until the oats and pecan pieces are completely coated.

3.   Spread the mixture on the baking sheet in an even layer. Bake in the oven for 20 minutes, stirring once halfway through cooking.

4.   Allow to cool on the countertop for 30 minutes before serving.

Nutrition: Calories: 221 Fat: 17.2g Carbs: 5.1g Protein: 4.9g Fiber: 3.8g

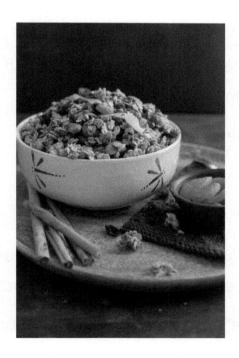

Herby Giant Couscous with Asparagus and Lemon

Servings: 2

Ingredients:

150 g giant couscous

100 g asparagus

110 g peas

3 and half tbsp. oil

Juice and zest of 1 lemon Handful fresh parsley Handful of fresh mint Handful baby spinach

2 tbsp. pine nuts

Directions:

1.   Add giant couscous to water. After 5 minutes, add asparagus and peas and boil for another 4 minutes.

2.   While the couscous is cooking, cooking in a mini blender (or directly in a bowl, sharp knife, elbow grease!), Walnut oil, lemon juice, parsley, and mint.

3. Drain the couscous and immediately stir the dressing of the baby herb and spinach.

4. Divide between two plates and crush with pine nuts and lemon lotion.

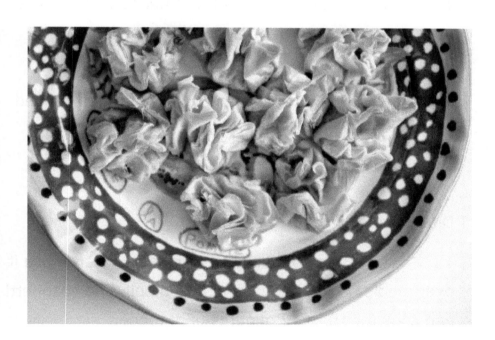

Tomato Basil Spaghetti

Preparation Time: 5 minutes

Cooking Time: 20 minutes

Servings: 4

Ingredients:

15-   ounce cooked great northern beans 10.5-ounces cherry tomatoes, halved 1 small white onion, peeled, diced

1   tablespoon minced garlic 8 basil leaves, chopped

2   tablespoons olive oil 1-pound spaghetti

Directions:

1.   Take a large pot half full with salty water, place it over medium-high heat, bring it to a boil, add spaghetti and cook for 10 to 12 minutes until tender.

2.   Then drain spaghetti into a colander and reserve 1 cup of pasta liquid.

3.   Add oil on a skillet pan and when hot, add onion, tomatoes, basil, and garlic and cook for 5 minutes until vegetables have turned tender.

4.   Add cooked spaghetti and beans, pour in pasta water, stir until just mixed and cook for 2 minutes until hot.

5.   Serve straight away.

Nutrition: 147 Cal 5 g Fat 0.7 g Saturated Fat 21.2 g Carbohydrates 1.5 g Fiber 5.4 g Sugars 3.8 g Protein;

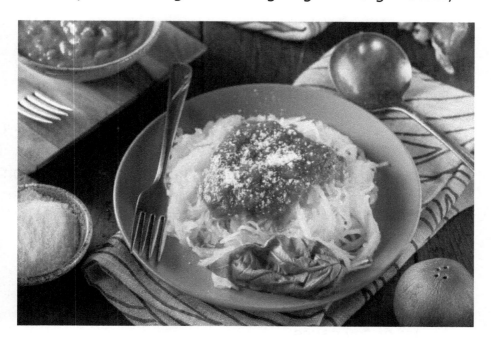

Jamaican Jerk Tofu Wrap

Preparation Time: 1 hour and 15 minutes

Cooking Time: 16 minutes

Servings: 4

Ingredients:

28 ounces tofu, firmed, pressed, drain, ½-inch long sliced

For the Marinade:

2 small scotch bonnet pepper, deseeded, minced 2 teaspoons minced garlic

2 1/2 teaspoons sea salt 4 teaspoons allspice

2 teaspoon ground black pepper 4 teaspoons cinnamon

4 teaspoons maple syrup 4 teaspoons nutmeg

4 tablespoons apple cider vinegar

2 teaspoon avocado oil and more for cooking

½ cup of soy sauce

2 tablespoon tomato paste For the Wrap:

4 cups baby spinach leaves

2 small tomato, deseeded, diced

2 medium yellow bell pepper, deseeded, cut into strips
4 tablespoons Sriracha sauce

4 tortillas, whole-grain

Directions:

1.   Place in a bowl all the ingredients for the marinade in it, whisk until combined, then add tofu pieces, toss until well coated, and let it marinate for a minimum of 1 hour, turning halfway.

2.   Add to a pan some of the avocado oil, and when hot, add tofu pieces and cook for 7 and half minutes per side until caramelized.

3.   Assemble the wrap and for this, place a tortilla on clean working space, top with 1 cup of spinach, half of each diced tomatoes and pepper strips, then top with 4 strips of tofu, drizzle with Sriracha sauce and wrap tightly.

4.   Repeat with the remaining tortilla, then cut each tortilla in half and serve.

Nutrition: 250 Cal 6 g Fat 1 g Saturated Fat 40 g
Carbohydrates 7 g Fiber 11 g Sugars 9 g Protein;

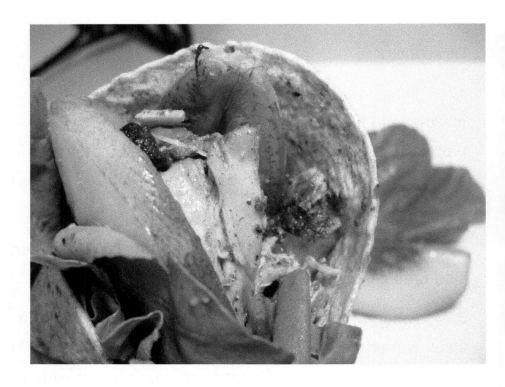

Bean and Rice Burritos

Preparation Time: 10 minutes

Cooking Time: 20 minutes

Servings: 6

Ingredients:

32 ounces refried beans 2 cups cooked rice

2 cups chopped spinach 1 tablespoon olive oil 1/2 cup tomato salsa

6 tortillas, whole-grain, warm Guacamole as needed for serving

Directions:

1.   Set the oven to 365 degrees F and let it preheat.

2.   Place a saucepan over medium heat, add beans, and cook for 3 to 5 minutes until softened; remove the pan from heat.

3. Place one tortilla in a clean working space, spread some of the beans on it into a log, leaving 2-inches of the edge, top beans with spinach, rice, and salsa, and then tightly wrap the tortilla to seal the filling like a burrito.

4. Repeat with the remaining tortillas, place these burritos on a baking sheet, brush them with olive oil and then bake for 15 minutes until golden.

5. Serve burritos with guacamole.

Nutrition: 421 Cal 9 g Fat 2 g Saturated Fat 70 g Carbohydrates 11 g Fiber 3 g Sugars 15 g Protein;

Chickpea Curry Soup

Preparation Time: 5 minutes

Cooking Time: 12 minutes

Servings: 4

Ingredients:

2 cups cooked chickpeas

1/4 of a medium white onion, peeled, chopped 1 tablespoon minced garlic

1 teaspoon ground coriander

¼ teaspoon cayenne pepper

1 tbsp curry powder

1 teaspoon turmeric

½ of a lime, juiced

1   tablespoon olive oil 2/3 cup coconut cream 2 cups vegetable broth

2   tablespoons pumpkin seeds

Directions:

1.   Place a saucepan over medium-high heat, add oil, and when hot.

2.   Add chickpeas, sprinkle with all the spices, stir until mixed and continue cooking for 5 minutes.

3.   Pour in vegetable broth, simmer for 5 minutes, then stir in cream, lime juice and remove the pan from heat.

4.   Ladle soup into bowls, top with pumpkin seeds, and then serve.

Nutrition: 154 Cal 8 g Fat 1 g Saturated Fat 16.5 g Carbohydrates 4 g Fiber

3   g Sugars 4.5 g Protein;

Roasted Green Beans

Preparation Time: 5 minutes

Cooking Time: 25 minutes

Servings: 2

Ingredients:

½ pound green beans

½ cup grated parmesan cheese 3 tablespoons coconut oil

½ teaspoon garlic powder

Extra:

1/3 teaspoon salt

1/8 teaspoon ground black pepper

Directions:

1.   Put the oven to 415 degrees F, and let preheat.

2.   Take a baking sheet, line green beans on it, and set aside until required.

3.   Prepare the dressing, and for this, place the remaining ingredients in a bowl, except for cheese, and whisk until combined.

4.   Drizzle the dressing over green beans, toss until well coated, and then bake for 20 minutes until green beans are tender-crisp.

5.   Then sprinkle cheese on top of beans and continue roasting for 3 to 5 minutes or until cheese melts and nicely golden brown.

6.   Serve straight away.

Nutrition: calories 119 fat 5 carbs 3 protein 8

Falafel Wrap

Total time: 70 minutes

Ingredients:

For the Falafel Patties

1   chickpeas, drained and rinsed, or 1½ cups cooked

1 zucchini, grated

2   scallions, minced

¼ cup fresh parsley, chopped

2 tablespoons black olives, pitted and chopped (optional)

1 tablespoon tahini, or almond, cashew, or sunflower seed butter

1 tbsp lemon juice

½ teaspoon ground cumin

¼ teaspoon paprika

¼ teaspoon sea salt

1 teaspoon olive oil (optional, if frying)

For the wrap

1 whole-grain wrap or pita

¼ cup Classic Hummus

½ cup fresh greens 1 baked falafel patty

¼ cup cherry tomatoes halved

¼ cup diced cucumber

¼ cup chopped avocado, or Guacamole

¼ cup cooked quinoa, or Tabbouleh Salad (optional)

Directions:

For the Falafel

1.   Mix chickpeas, zucchini, scallions, parsley, and olives (if using) until roughly chopped. Just pulse—don't purée. Put the chickpeas in a bowl and stir in the grated and chopped veggies.

2.   Whisk the tahini and lemon juice, and stir in the cumin, paprika, and salt. Pour this into the chickpea mixture, and stir well (or pulse the food processor) to combine. Taste and add more salt, if needed. Form the mix into 6 patties.

3.   You can either panfry or bake the patties. To panfry, heat a large skillet to medium, add 1 teaspoon of olive oil, and cook the patties for about 10 minutes on the first side. Flip and cook for another 5 to 7 minutes. Bake at 340°F for 35 minutes.

Directions for the wrap:

1.   Spread the hummus down the center. Then lay on the greens and crumble the falafel patty on top. Add the tomatoes, cucumber, avocado, and quinoa.

2.   Press the wraps for about 5 minutes.

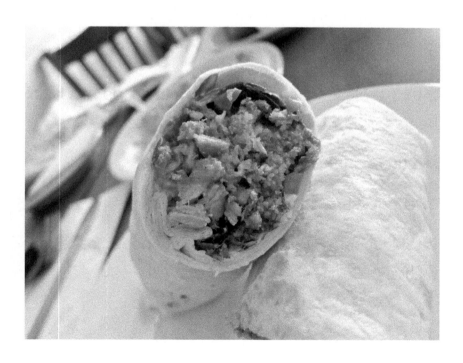

Pad Thai Bowl

Total time: 20 minutes

Ingredients:

7 ounces brown rice noodles

1 tsp olive oil, or 1 tablespoon vegetable

2 carrots, peeled or scrubbed, and julienned

1   cup thinly sliced napa cabbage, or red cabbage 1 red bell pepper, seeded and thinly sliced

2   scallions, finely chopped

2 to 3 tablespoons fresh mint, finely chopped 1 cup bean sprouts

¼ cup Peanut Sauce

¼ cup fresh cilantro, finely chopped

2 tablespoons roasted peanuts, chopped Fresh lime wedges

Directions:

1.   Cover rice noodles with boiling water. Let sit until they soften, about 10 minutes. Rinse, drain, and set aside to cool.

2.   Sauté the carrots, cabbage, and bell pepper until softened, 7 to 8 minutes. Toss in the scallions, mint, and bean sprouts and cook for just a minute or two, then remove from the heat.

3.   Toss the noodles with the vegetables, and mix in the Peanut Sauce.

4.   Transfer to bowls, and sprinkle with cilantro and peanuts. Serve with a lime wedge to squeeze onto the dish for a flavor boost.

5.   Options: To enjoy an even more nutrient-dense version of this bowl, leave out the rice noodles and peel or spiralize zucchini or carrot into long "noodles."

Curry Spiced Lentil Burgers

Total time: 80 minutes

Ingredients:

1 cup lentils

2½ to 3 cups water 3 carrots, grated

1 small onion, diced

¾ cup whole-grain flour (see Options for gluten-free below) 1½ to 2 teaspoons curry powder

½ teaspoon sea salt

Pinch freshly ground black pepper

Directions:

1.   Put the lentils in water. Boil and then simmer for 33 minutes, until soft.

2.   Put carrots and onion in a bowl. Toss them with flour, curry powder, salt, and pepper.

3.   Drain off any excess water, then add them to the veggies bowl. Add more flour if you need to get the mixture to stick together. The amount of flour depends on how much water the lentils absorbed and the flour's texture, so use more or less until the mixture sticks when you form it into a ball. Scoop up ¼-cup portions and form into 12 patties.

4.   You can either panfry or bake the burgers. To panfry, heat a large skillet to medium, add a tiny bit of oil, and cook the burgers for about 10 minutes on the first side. Flip and cook for another 5 to 7 minutes. Bake at 340°F for 35 minutes.

5.   Options: For the whole-grain flour, use whatever flour you like. Sorghum, rice, oat, buckwheat, and even almond meal would work and make these gluten-free. The flour in this recipe is just a binding agent so that it can be any type.

Black Bean Taco Salad Bowl

Total time: 20 minutes

Ingredients

For the Black Bean Salad

1 (14-ounce) can black beans,

1 cup corn kernels

¼ cup cilantro, chopped

juice of 1 lime

1 to 2 teaspoons chili powder Pinch sea salt

1½ cups tomatoes

1 pepper, seeded and chopped

2 scallions, chopped

For 1 Serving of Tortilla Chips

1 sizeable whole-grain tortilla

1 teaspoon olive oil

Pinch sea salt

Pinch freshly ground black pepper Pinch dried oregano

Pinch chili powder

For 1 Bowl

1   cup fresh greens (lettuce, spinach, or whatever you like)

¾ cup cooked quinoa, or brown rice, millet, or other whole grain

¼ cup chopped avocado, or Guacamole

¼ cup Fresh Mango Salsa

Directions for the salad

Toss all the ingredients in a bowl.

Directions

1.   for the tortilla chips

2.   Brush the tortilla with olive oil, then sprinkle with salt, pepper, oregano, chili powder, and any other seasonings you like. Transfer the tortilla pieces to a small baking sheet lined with parchment paper and put in the oven or toaster oven to toast or broil for 3 to 5

minutes, until browned. Keep an eye on them, as they can go from just barely done to burned very quickly.

Directions for the bowl

1.   Put the greens in the bowl, top with the cooked quinoa, ⅓ of the black bean salad, the avocado, and salsa.

2.   The black bean mixture tastes better if you make it in advance, so the flavors have time to mix and mingle. Keep leftovers in the fridge in an airtight container.

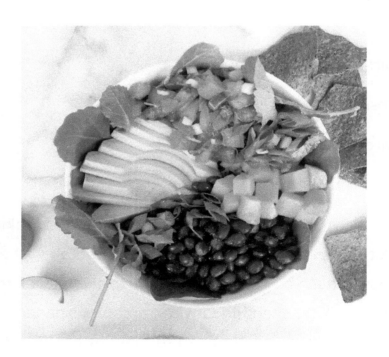

Bibimbap Bowl

Total time: 30 minutes

Ingredients

½ cup cooked chickpeas

2   tablespoons tamari or soy sauce, divided

1 tablespoon plus 2 teaspoons toasted sesame oil, divided

¾ cup cooked brown rice, or quinoa, millet, or any other whole grain

1   tsp olive oil

1 carrot, scrubbed or peeled, and julienned

2   garlic cloves, minced, divided Pinch sea salt

½ cup asparagus, cut into 2-inch pieces

 ½ cup chopped spinach

½ cup bean sprouts

3   tablespoons hot pepper paste (the Korean version is gochujang) 1 tablespoon toasted sesame seeds

1 scallion, chopped

Directions

1.   Toss the chickpeas with 1 tablespoon tamari and 1 teaspoon toasted sesame oil. Set aside to marinate.

2.   Put rice in a serving bowl so that you'll be ready to add the vegetables as they cook.

3.   Heat the olive oil a large skillet over medium heat, and start by sautéing the carrot and 1 garlic clove with the salt. Once they've softened, about 5 minutes, remove them from the skillet and put them on top of the rice in one area of the bowl.

4.   Next, sauté the asparagus, adding a bit more oil if necessary, and when soft, about 5 minutes, place next to the carrots in the bowl.

5.   Add a bit of water to the skillet and quick steam the spinach with the other garlic clove, just until the spinach wilts. Drizzle with the remaining 1 tablespoon tamari and 1 teaspoon toasted sesame oil. Lay the spinach on the other side of the carrots in the bowl.

6. You could lightly sauté the bean sprouts if you wish, but they're excellent raw. However you prefer them, add them to the bowl.

7. 7.Place the marinated chickpeas in the final area of the bowl.

8. In a small bowl, mix the hot pepper paste with 1 tablespoon sesame oil. Scoop that into the middle of the bowl. Sprinkle with sesame seeds and scallions, then mix it all and enjoy!

Colcannon-Topped Vegan Shepherds' Pie

Servings: 6

Ingredients:

For the Pie Filling

1 and half carrot

1 potato

2 tbsp. rapeseed or sunflower oil

1 onion

400 g tin cannellini beans

400 g tin green or brown lentils

400 g tin chopped tomatoes

1 tsp vegetable stock powder (check it is vegan)

2 tbsp. gravy granules (check they are vegan) For the Colcannon Mash

600 g potatoes

60 g curly kale

3 spring onions

50 ml dairy-free milk (soy, oat, or nut milk)

20 g dairy-free margarine

Directions:

1. Heat the oven to 180 degrees Celsius.

2. Boil a large pot of water. Meanwhile, peel the sweet carrots and potatoes and smooth them. Simmer for 10 minutes

3. Also, heat the oil in a large bowl or a large bowl with the pan, chop and add to the pan, fry over low heat for 3-4 minutes.

4. Wash and wash beans and lentils and add onions with tomatoes, broth powder, and gravitational seeds. Fill the empty tomato can with water, fill approximately two-thirds of it, and then add it to the pot.

5. When the carrots and sweet potatoes are freshly cooked, remove them with a slotted spoon and add them to the cake filling (do not waste water yet!). Cook and cover, and simmer for 9 minutes. If the mixture becomes too dry, add more water; It should have a

thick consistency of fat. (And if it also seems climatic, cook for a few minutes with the lid on.)

6.   Stir the pot until the potatoes are peeled, cut them into cubes, then add them to the pan and cook for 10-15 minutes.

7.   Meanwhile, cut the chives stalks as much as possible. Add the cabbage, chives, milk, and margarine and cook until they are uniform.

8.   Disinfect the stuffed leg in a large bowl, then cover with mashed potatoes. I used a plumbing bag to create a beautiful summit.

9.   Bake for 32 minutes until it is soft, golden, and full of bubbles.

Vegan Sausage Casserole: Bangers & Borlotti Bean Stew

Servings: 3

Ingredients:

2 tbsp. olive or rapeseed oil

6 vegan sausages

1 red onion

8 baby carrots (e.g., chantey)

1 tsp smoked paprika

1 tsp garlic puree Protein content per serving

410 g borlotti beans (drained and rinsed)

250 g passata

2 tbsp. gravy granules (check they are vegan)

handful baby spinach

Instructions:

1.   Fry the oil in a large pan and fry the sausages over medium heat to brown. Addthe onion to the pot,

then finely chop the carrots and cut them in half or a quarter. Cook for 3 and half minutes.

2.   Add the garlic to onion and paprika to the pot and stir well. Rinse and wash the Borlotti beans, add them to the pan, and add 250 ml of water and gravitational seeds. Reduce to medium heat and cook for 7-8 minutes until the sauce thickens and the carrots are well prepared. Add some salt or black pepper if necessary and try.

3.   Chop the spinach almost and stir only one minute before the end of the cooking time. Serve with a baked potato, rice, or noodles.

Protein Content Per Servings: 21.7g

BBQ Black Bean & Jalepeño Burger

Servings: 6 burgers

Ingredients:

2 x 410g black beans, drained and rinsed 4 spring onions

12-14 slices jalapeno

175 g breadcrumbs Juice and zest of 1 lime

2 tsp ready chopped garlic Protein content per serving garlic puree

Handful fresh coriander, finely chopped

2 tbsp. soy sauce

2 tbsp. tahini

Salt & black pepper

Directions:

1.   Put the black beans in a food processor and press several times until it is crushed but not wholly purified.

(Alternatively, break them with potato sand). Pour into a large bowl.

2.   Chop the scallions and finely chop the slices. Add both to the bowl, followed by breadcrumbs, lemon zest and juice, garlic, coriander, soy sauce, and Tahini. Season with salt and pepper.

3.   Mix the ingredients to combine well, then divide them into approximately 5-6 pieces (or for smaller burgers 7-8). Use your hamburger machine or shape hamburgers by hand, then place them on a cooked tray covered with baking paper and refrigerate for as long as necessary.

4.   To grill: rinse each side with a little oil and cook for 5 minutes in the oven

5.   On the clock

6.   For cooking: Brush each side with oil and bake at 190 degrees Celsius at 375 degrees Fahrenheit for 5 minutes for 20 minutes.

7.   To fry: fry in oil for 5 minutes on each side.

8.   Serve with chopped avocado, tomato slices, lettuce, purple onion, gherkins, or a slice of cheese and dairy-free tomato sauce.

Slow Cooker Butternut Dhal

Servings: 4

Ingredients:

1   red onion

2   tbsp. rapeseed or sunflower oil

1 tsp garlic puree Protein content per serving ready-chopped garlic

1 tsp ginger puree Protein content per serving ready-chopped ginger

1 red chili,

4 tsp curry powder

210 g lentils, rinsed

410 ml coconut milk

1 tsp vegetable stock powder

300 g butternut squash

To finish:

1 lemon

1 green chili handful fresh coriander

Directions:

To build a Redmond Multicooker:

1.   Chop and chop the onion and place it in a pot with oil, garlic, ginger, pepper, and powder. Cook for 5 minutes in the FRY setting, stirring occasionally.

2.   Add lentils, coconut milk, refill the empty can with water and add this, followed by powdered broth. Peel the butternut squash, pour it into small cubes (approximately 1 cm), and add it to the mixture. Serve the season with salt and pepper. Cook slowly in the kitchen for 2 hours, occasionally stirring until the lentils soften and the dhal has a creamy consistency. Check and adjust seasoning and then serve.

3.   Heat 2 tbps of oil in a small pan to bake optionally. Chop the oilseeds and chop finely and add to the pot. Cook over medium-low heat until crispy. Spoon on the dial. Chop the cilantro and sprinkle on it, then finish with a little lemon juice.

To make a slow cooker:

4.   Chop and chop the onion and sprinkle with oil, garlic, garlic, ginger, pepper, and curry powder in a pan. Cook for 3 and half minutes, stirring occasionally.

5.   Pour slowly into the oven, then add the lentils and coconut milk. Fill the empty can again with water and add this, followed by powdered broth. Peel the butternut squash, pour it into small cubes (approximately 1 cm), and add it to the mixture. Serve the season with salt and pepper. Cook for 4 hours (or less than 8 hours) until the lentils soften and the dhal has a thick and creamy consistency. Check and adjust seasoning and then serve.

6.   Chop the oilseeds and chop finely and add to the pot. Cook over medium-low heat until crispy. Spoon on the dial. Chop the cilantro and sprinkle on it, then finish with a little lemon juice.

Spiced Tomato Brown Rice

Preparation Time: 10 minutes

Cooking Time: 15 minutes

Servings: 4 to 6

Ingredients:

1 onion

1 green bell pepper

3 cloves garlic, minced

¼ cup water

15 to 16oz. (425 to 454g) tomatoes, chopped 1 tablespoon chili powder

2 tsp ground cumin

1 tsp dried basil

½ teaspoon Parsley Patch seasoning, general blend

¼ teaspoon cayenne

2 cups cooked brown rice

Directions:

1.   Combine the onion, green pepper, garlic, and water in a saucepan over medium heat. Cook for 4 minutes, stirring frequently, or until softened.

2.   Add the tomatoes and seasonings. Cook for another 5 minutes. Stir in the cooked rice. Cook for another 4 and half minutes to allow the flavors to blend.

3.   Serve immediately.

Nutrition: Calories: 107 Fat: 1.1g Carbs: 21.1g Protein: 3.2g

Fiber: 2.9g

Noodle and Rice Pilaf

Preparation Time: 5 minutes

Cooking Time: 33 to 44 minutes

Servings: 6 to 8

Ingredients:

1 cup whole-wheat noodles, broken into 1/8 inch pieces

2 cups long-grain brown rice

6½ cups vegetable broth

1 tsp ground cumin

½ teaspoon dried oregano

Directions:

1.   Combine the noodles and rice in a saucepan over medium heat and cook for 3 to 4 minutes, or until they begin to smell toasted.

2.   Stir in the vegetable broth, cumin, and oregano. Bring to a boil. Reduce the heat to medium-low. Cover and cook for 33 minutes, or until all water is absorbed.

Nutrition:

Calories: 287 Fat: 2.5g Carbs: 58.1g Protein: 7.9g Fiber: 5.0g

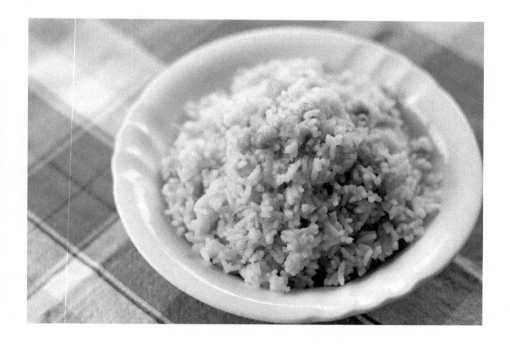

Easy Millet Loaf

Preparation Time: 5 minutes

Cooking Time: 1 hour 15 minutes

Servings: 4

Ingredients:

1¼ cups millet

4 cups unsweetened tomato juice 1 medium onion, chopped

1 to 2 cloves garlic

½ teaspoon dried sage

½ teaspoon dried basil

½ teaspoon poultry seasoning

Directions:

1.   Preheat the oven to 350ºF.

2.   Place the millet in a large bowl.

3.   Place the remaining ingredients in a blender and pulse until smooth. Add to the bowl with the millet and mix well.

4.   Pour the mixture into a shallow casserole dish. Cover and bake in the oven for 1¼ hours or until set.

5.   Serve warm.

Nutrition:

Calories: 315 Fat: 3.4g Carbs: 61.6g Protein: 10.2g Fiber: 9.6g

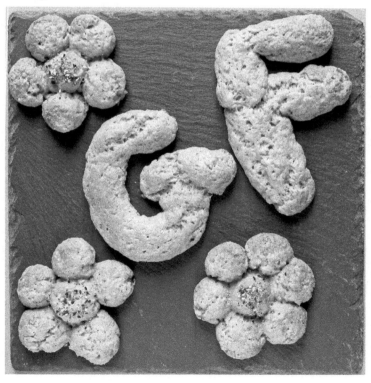

Walnut-Oat Burgers

Preparation Time: 5 minutes

Cooking Time: 20 to 30 minutes

Servings: 6 to 8

Ingredients:

1   medium onion, finely chopped 2 cups rolled oats

2   cups unsweetened low-Fat: soy milk 1 cup finely chopped walnuts

1 tablespoon soy sauce

½ teaspoon dried sage

½ teaspoon garlic powder

½ teaspoon onion powder

½ teaspoon dried thyme

¼ teaspoon dried marjoram

Directions:

1.   Stir together all the ingredients in a large bowl. Let rest for 20 minutes.

2.   Form the mixture into six or eight patties. Cook the patties on a nonstick skillet over medium heat for 20 to 30 minutes or until browned on each side.

3.   Serve warm.

Nutrition:

Calories: 341 Fat: 13.9g Carbs: 42.4g Protein: 13.9g Fiber: 6.8g

Beans and Rice

Preparation Time: 5 minutes

Cooking Time: 45 minutes

Servings: 4 to 6

Ingredients:

1½ cups long-grain brown rice

1 (19-oz.) can kidney beans, rinsed and drained 2 cups chopped onion

1 cup mild salsa

1 teaspoon ground cumin 16 oz. tomatoes, chopped 3 cups water

Directions:

1.   In a pot, bring the water to a boil. Stir in the rice. Bring to a boil again and stir in the remaining ingredients, except for the tomatoes. Return to a boil. Reduce the heat to low. Cover and simmer for 45 minutes.

2.   Remove from the heat and stir in the tomatoes. Let sit for 5 minutes, covered.

Nutrition: Calories: 386 Fat: 7.1g Carbs: 71.1g

Protein: 11.1g Fiber: 5.8g

Vegan Alfredo Fettuccine Pasta

Preparation Time: 15 minutes

Cooking Time: 15 minutes

Servings: 1

Ingredients:

White potatoes - 2 medium White onion - ¼

Italian seasoning - 1 tablespoon

Lemon juice - 1 teaspoon Garlic - 2 cloves

Salt - 1 teaspoon

Fettuccine pasta - 12 ounces Raw cashew - ½ cup

Nutritional yeast (optional) - 1 teaspoon Truffle oil (optional) - ¼ teaspoon

Directions:

1.   Start by placing a pot on high flame and boiling 4 cups of water.

2.   Peel the potatoes and cut them into small cubes. Cut the onion into cubes as well.

3.   Add the potatoes and onions to the boiling water and cook for about 10 minutes.

4.   Remove the onions and potatoes. Keep aside. Save the water.

5. Season generously with salt.

6.   Toss in the fettuccine pasta and cook as per package instructions.

7.   Take a blender and add in the raw cashews, veggies, nutritional yeast, truffle oil, lemon juice, and 1 cup of the saved water. Blend into a smooth puree.

8.   Add in the garlic and salt.

9.   Drain the cooked pasta using a colander. Transfer into a mixing bowl.

10.   Serve.

Nutrition: calories 884 fat 13 carbs 15 protein 6

Spinach Pasta in Pesto Sauce

Preparation Time: 20 minutes

Cooking Time: 15 minutes

Servings: 1

Ingredients:

 Olive oil - 1 tablespoon Spinach - 5 ounces

All-purpose flour - 2 cups

Salt - 1 tablespoon plus ¼ teaspoon (keep it divided)
Water - 2 tablespoons

Roasted vegetable for serving Pesto for serving

Fresh basil for serving

Directions:

1.   Place a pot with water over a high flame and bring the water to a boil. Add one tablespoon of salt

2.   Place a saucepan over a medium flame. Put on the olive oil and heat it through.

3. Toss in the spinach and sauté for 5 minutes.

4. Take a food processor and transfer the wilted spinach. Process until the spinach is delicate in texture.

5. Add in the flour and continue to process to form a crumbly dough.

6. Further, add ¼ teaspoon of salt and 1 tbsp of water while processing to bring the dough together.

7. Sprinkle dough with flour. Knead well to form a dough ball.

8. Roll out the dough. The dimensions of the rolled dough should be 18 inches long and 12 inches wide. The thickness should be about ¼ - inch thick.

9. Cut the rolled dough into long and even strips using a pizza cutter. Make sure the strips are ½ - inch wide.

10. The strips need to be rolled into evenly sized thick noodles.

11. Toss in the prepared noodles and cook for about 4 minutes. Drain using a colander.

12. Transfer the noodles into a large mixing bowl and add in the roasted vegetables, pesto. Toss well to combine.

13. Garnish with basil leaves.

Nutrition: calories 591 fat 8 carbs 42 protein 16

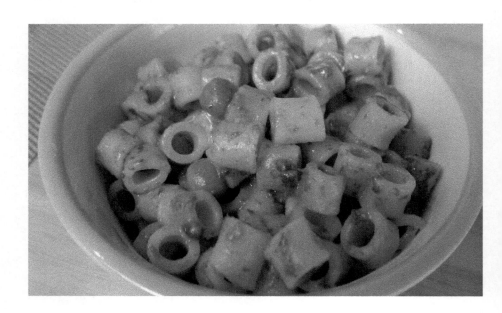

Creamy Curry Noodles

Preparation Time: 19 minutes

Cooking Time: 10 minutes

Servings: 4

Ingredients:

Creamy Curry Sauce

Apple cider vinegar, two tablespoons Water, one-quarter of one cup Avocado oil, two tablespoons Turmeric, ground, one teaspoon Black pepper, one half teaspoon Tahini, one-quarter of one cup

Coriander, ground, one- and one-half teaspoons Cumin, ground, one teaspoon

Salt, one teaspoon

Curry powder, two teaspoons Ginger, ground, one quarter teaspoon

Noodle Bowl

Cilantro, fresh, chopped small, one half cup Bell pepper, red, one cleaned and diced Zucchini noodles, one sixteen-ounce pack Carrots, two, peeled and cut in julienne strips Kale, two cups packed

Cauliflower, one half of one head chopped small

Directions:

1.   Cover the zucchini noodles with two cups of boiling water in a medium-sized bowl and set them off to the side. After leaving the noodles in the water for five minutes, drain off the water and place them back into the bowl. Prep all of the veggies and then toss them into the bowl with the noodles. Toss the ingredients in the bowl gently, but okay.

2.   Divide the leaves of kale onto four serving plates. Mix the list of ingredients for the Creamy Curry Sauce and blend them until they are smooth and creamy. When the sauce is well mixed, then pour it over the ingredients in the bowl and toss the ingredients well until all are covered with the sauce.

3.   Then divide the noodles over the kale on the four plates and serve.

Roasted Vegetables

Preparation Time: 10 minutes

Cooking Time: 20 minutes

Servings: 4

Ingredients:

Cilantro, chopped, one-quarter of one cup Green onion, diced, one half of one cup

Masala Seasoning

Black pepper, one half teaspoon Turmeric, one quarter teaspoon

Chili powder, ground, one half teaspoon Tomato puree, one half of one cup Garam masala, one quarter teaspoon salt, one half teaspoon

Garlic, minced, one tablespoon Olive oil, two tablespoons Ginger, ground, two teaspoons

Veggies

Cauliflower, one cup in small pieces

Mushrooms sliced one half of one cup Green beans, three-fourths of one cup

Directions:

1.   Heat the oven to 400. Place the rack in the oven in the middle. Use aluminum foil or parchment paper to cover a baking sheet completely. Use a medium-sized bowl to mix the chili powder, ginger, garam masala, garlic, pepper, salt, and tomato puree, making sure the ingredients are all mixed well.

2.   Then mix in the olive oil. Place the chopped veggies into this mixture and mix them in well. Then place the coated veggies onto the covered baking sheet in one single layer.

3.   Roast the veggies in the heated oven for thirty to forty minutes or until the veggies are cooked in a manner you like them.

Nutrition: calories 105 fat 10 carbs 13 protein 3

Delicious Broccoli

Preparation Time: 15 minutes

Cooking Time: 15 minutes

Servings: 8

Ingredients:

2 oranges, sliced in half 1 lb. broccoli rabe

2 tablespoons sesame oil, toasted Salt, and pepper to taste

1 tablespoon sesame seeds, toasted

Directions:

1.   Put the oil on a pan.

2.   Add the oranges and cook until caramelized.

3.   Transfer to a plate.

4.   Put the broccoli in the pan and cook for 8 minutes.

5.   Squeeze the oranges to release juice in a bowl.

6.   Stir in the oil, salt, and pepper.

7.   Coat the broccoli rabe with the mixture.

8.   Sprinkle seeds on top.

Nutrition: calories 432 fat 1 carbs 24 protein 12

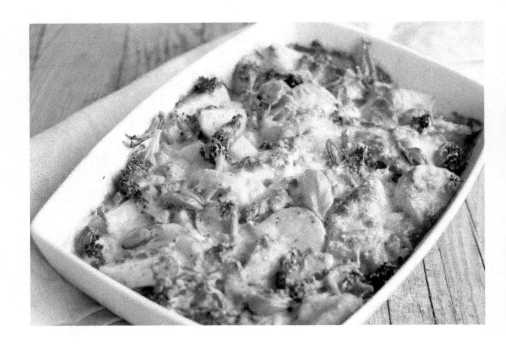

Spicy Peanut Soba Noodles

Preparation Time: 7 minutes

Cooking Time: 17 minutes

Servings: 1

Ingredients:

5 ounces uncooked soba noodles

½ tablespoon low sodium soy sauce 1 clove garlic, minced

4 teaspoons water

1 small head of broccoli, cut into florets

½ cup carrot

¼ cup finely chopped scallions 3 tablespoons peanut butter

1 tablespoon honey

1 teaspoon crushed red pepper flakes 2 teaspoons vegetable oil

4 ounces button mushrooms, discard stems 3 tablespoons peanuts, dry roasted, unsalted

Directions:

1.   Cook soba noodles as the directions on the package says.

2.   Add peanut butter, honey, water, soy sauce, garlic, and red pepper flakes. Whisk until well combined.

3.   Place a skillet over medium heat. Add oil. When the oil is heated, add broccoli and sauté for a few minutes until crisp as well as tender.

4.   Add mushrooms and sauté until the mushrooms are tender. Turn off the heat.

5.   Add the sauce mixture and carrots and mix well.

6.   Crush the peanuts by rolling with a rolling pin.

7.   Divide the noodles into bowls. Pour sauce mixture over it.

Nutrition: calories 512 fat 11 carbs 20 protein 8

Grilled Ahlt

Total time: 15 minutes

Ingredients:

¼ cup Classic Hummus

2 slices whole-grain bread

¼ avocado, sliced

½ cup lettuce, chopped

½ tomato, sliced Pinch sea salt

Pinch freshly pepper

1 tsp olive oil, divided

Directions:

1.   Spread some hummus on each slice of bread. Then layer the avocado, lettuce, and tomato on one slice, sprinkle with salt and pepper and top with the other slice.

2.   Drizzle ½ teaspoon of olive oil just before putting the sandwich in the skillet. Cook for 3 to 5 minutes, then lift the sandwich with a spatula, drizzle the remaining

½ teaspoon olive oil into the skillet, and flip the sandwich to grill the other side for 3 5 minutes. Press it down with the spatula to seal the vegetables inside.

3.   Once done, remove from the skillet and slice in half to serve.

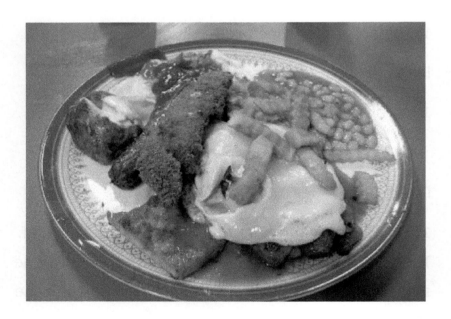

Loaded Black Bean Pizza

Total time: 30 minutes

Ingredients:

2 prebaked pizza crusts

½ cup Spicy Black Bean Dip

1 tomato, thinly sliced

Pinch freshly ground black pepper 1 carrot, grated

Pinch sea salt

1 red onion, thinly sliced 1 avocado, sliced

Directions:

1.   Preheat the oven to 400°F.

2.   Lay the two crusts out on a large baking sheet. Spread half the Spicy Black Bean Dip on each pizza crust. Then layer on the tomato slices with a pinch of pepper if you like.

3.   Sprinkle the grated carrot with the sea salt and lightly massage it in with your hands. Spread the carrot on top of the tomato, then add the onion.

4.   Pop the pizzas in the oven for 10 to 20 minutes or until they're done to your taste.

5.   Top the cooked pizzas with sliced avocado and another sprinkle of pepper.

6.   Options: Try having this as a fresh unbaked pizza. Just toast a pita or bake the crust before loading it up, and perhaps use scallions instead of red. Bonus points— and flavor—if you top it with fresh alfalfa sprouts.

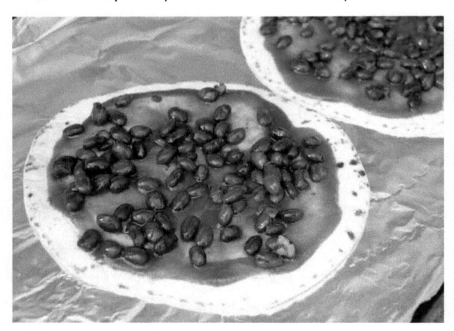

Brown Rice with Mushrooms

Preparation Time: 15 minutes

Cooking Time: 20 minutes

Servings: 6 to 8

Ingredients:

½ pound (227 g) mushrooms, sliced 1 green bell pepper, chopped

1 onion

1 bunch scallions

2 cloves garlic, minced

½ cup water

5 cups cooked brown rice

1 (16-oz. / 454-g) can chopped tomatoes

1 (4-oz. / 113-g) can chop green chilies 2 teaspoons chili powder

1 teaspoon ground cumin

Directions:

1.   In a large pot, sauté the mushrooms, green pepper, onion, scallions, and garlic in the water for 10 minutes.

2.   Stir in the remaining ingredients. Cook for 7 and half minutes or until heated through, stirring frequently.

3.   Serve immediately.

Nutrition:

Calories: 185 Fat: 2.6g Carbs: 34.5g Protein: 6.1g Fiber: 4.3g

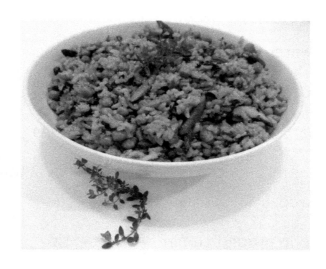

Veggie Paella

Preparation Time: 15 minutes

Cooking Time: 52 to 58 minutes

Servings: 4

Ingredients:

1 onion, coarsely chopped

8 medium mushrooms, sliced

2 small zucchinis, cut in half, then sliced ½ inch thick 1 leek, rinsed, and sliced

2 large cloves garlic, crushed

1 medium tomato, coarsely chopped 3 cups low-sodium vegetable broth 1¼ cups long-grain brown rice

½ teaspoon crushed saffron threads Freshly ground black pepper, to taste

½ cup frozen green peas

½ cup water

Chopped fresh parsley for garnish

Directions:

1.   Pour the water in a large wok. Add the onion and sauté for 4 and half minutes, or until most of the liquid is absorbed.

2.   Stir in the mushrooms, zucchini, leek, and garlic, cook for 2 to 3 minutes, or soften slightly.

3.   Add the tomato, broth, rice, saffron, and pepper. Bring to a boil. Cook for 30 minutes.

4.   Let rest for 9 minutes to allow any excess moisture to be absorbed.

5.   Sprinkle with the parsley before serving.

Nutrition:

Calories: 418 Fat: 3.9g Carbs: 83.2g Protein: 12.7g Fiber: 9.2g

Vegetable and Wild Rice Pilaf

Preparation Time: 10 minutes

Cooking Time: 48 to 49 minutes

Servings: 6

Ingredients:

1 potato, scrubbed and chopped 1 cup chopped cauliflower

1 cup chopped scallion 1 cup chopped broccoli

1 to 2 cloves garlic, minced 2 tablespoons soy sauce

3 cups low-sodium vegetable broth 1 cup long-grain brown rice

1/3 cup wild rice

2 small zucchinis, chopped

½ cup grated carrot

1/8 teaspoon sesame oil (optional)

¼ cup chopped fresh cilantro

½ cup water

Directions:

1.   Add the potato, cauliflower, scallion, broccoli to water and garlic and sauté for 2 to 3 minutes.

2.   Add the soy sauce and cook for 2 minute. Add the vegetable broth, brown rice, and wild rice. Bring to a boil. Reduce the heat, cover, and cook for 15 minutes.

3.   Stir in the zucchinis. After another 15 minutes, stir in the carrot. Continue to cook for 15 minutes. Stir in the sesame oil (if desired) and cilantro.

4.   Serve immediately.

Nutrition:

Calories: 376 Fat: 3.6g Carbs: 74.5g Protein: 11.8g Fiber: 8.1g

Brown Rice with Spiced Vegetables

Preparation Time: 10 minutes

Cooking Time: 16 to 18 minutes

Servings: 6

Ingredients:

2 teaspoons grated fresh ginger 2 cloves garlic, crushed

½ cup water

¼ pound (113 g) green beans, trimmed and cut into 1-inch pieces 1 carrot, scrubbed and sliced

½ pound mushrooms, sliced

2 zucchinis, cut in half lengthwise and sliced 1 bunch scallions, cut into 1-inch pieces

4 cups cooked brown rice 3 tablespoons soy sauce

Directions:

1.   Place the ginger and garlic in a large pot with the water. Add the green beans and carrot and sauté for 3 minutes.

2.   Add the mushrooms and sauté for another 2 minutes. Stir in the zucchini and scallions. Reduce the heat. Cook for 7minutes, or until the vegetables are tender-crisp, stirring frequently.

3.   Stir in the rice and soy sauce. Cook over low heat for 5 minutes or until heated through.

4.   Serve warm.

Nutrition:

Calories: 205 Fat: 3.0g Carbs: 38.0g Protein: 6.4g Fiber:4.4g

Lightning Source UK Ltd.
Milton Keynes UK
UKHW022007030521
383075UK00003B/332